Treat Your Own Shoulder Labrum

First Edition

ISBN-13: 978-1515061441

ISBN-10: 1515061442

PRINTED IN THE UNITED STATES OF AMERICA

A huge thank you to everyone who helped me walk again and showed me what really works to fix chronic pain. And to Kirk Whitaker, I couldn't have done it without you!

Table of Contents

So you tore your shoulder labrum... Now what?

If you have been dealing with the pain of a torn shoulder labrum, you will be frustrated. The pain can be relentless and can be present for weeks on end. When you go to the doctor, all they suggest is surgery. The reason this is usually the only option is due to the fact that the labrum cannot magically re-attach itself to your scapula. When the labrum is torn, it is dangling off your scapula, and there is nothing besides surgery that will re-attach it. Many people that are fitness advocates may say "I hate surgery and I am not getting it done".... But then months go by... and you lose your upper body strength, and surgery starts to sound really nice.

I tore both of my shoulder labrums from coaching and training in gymnastics. I dealt with the pain on my left shoulder for about 2 years, and the pain on my right shoulder for 5 years. I also had a nerve disease at the time and I was unable to get the surgery at first (trying to walk with my nerve disease was more important than my torn labrums). I thought I would never be able to get the surgery due to complications with my nerve disease, so I tried literally every treatment available. After I fixed my nerve disease, I was finally able to have the surgery.

I found that I could control the pain with a few therapies. Understand that I did not "fix" the pain entirely, but I made it so I could live a comfortable life for the time being. The therapies that helped me were never mentioned by doctors, and my current goal is to help others that experience this pain and frustration.

I have helped thousands of people with my other books on how to fix chronic inflammatory injuries, but unlike inflammatory based injuries, fixing a shoulder labrum is impossible (without surgery). A lot of therapies available will waste your time and your money. No matter how much dedication/positive thinking/hope/vitamins and supplements you have available, they will not fix your labrum.

This book is an ultimate guide to alleviating your pain in the meantime, and how to increase your odds of having a successful surgery free of complications.

Fix your diet first

The therapies that help a torn labrum will work extremely well if you have an awesome diet. Also, when the time comes to eventually get the surgery done, you need a solid diet so that your body can heal fast, and properly. If you do not give your body the nutrients it needs, the injury will not heal properly. You have one chance at getting the surgery right. Make sure that your nutrient intake can enable your body to accommodate your injury/surgery.

Most "healthy eating" books all have the same information. Eat clean, wholesome, unprocessed, organic foods. The list below shows an ideal diet to speed up healing and reduce pain:

A good diet has:
- Raw Organic Fruits and Vegetables
- Raw Organic Oils
- Sprouted Organic Nuts and Seeds
- Organic animal products that do not emphasize the meat. Meat lacks nutrients. Bones/organs/brains/eggs/liver are extremely dense in nutrients
- Fermented Foods
- Herbs and Spices
- Unrefined sea salt. Celtic sea salt is ideal

A bad diet has:
- Processed foods of all kinds. This includes packaged foods that are not fresh, pasteurized juices, bread and pasta, most canned foods, frozen foods, microwave dinners, etc. This is not real food!
- Fake Oils: Hydrogenated/Partially Hydrogenated Oils. These do not belong inside humans.
- Refined Carbohydrates: Sugar, Glucose, Dextrose, High Fructose Corn Syrup and Fruit Juices. Just because it is "organic evaporated cane juice" does not mean it is healthy. (Agave syrup may be low glycemic, but it is high in glycemic load. Avoid all sweeteners except for stevia.)
- Dairy products. Cow's milk is for baby cows. Goat's milk is for baby goats. Human consumption of dairy products is illogical. It can cause changes in your hormones, and can leech minerals from your body. Avoid at all costs.
- Corn/Soy/Canola/Cottonseed/Safflower oils
- Grains/Flours/Gluten free flours/Rice

- Cooked oils. Coconut oil should be the only oil you cook with. Most oils, especially polyunsaturated oils, are extremely unhealthy to consume after you cook them. People think they are making a healthy choice by using olive oil. Olive oil is only health when it is raw. If you heat it up, it becomes toxic.
- Cooked vegetables. Raw is much healthier.
- Toxic water. Tap water is horrible for you and is not for human consumption!
- Synthetic vitamins. Bioavailability (how much you can absorb of a nutrient) is very low from synthetic vitamins. To absorb vitamins, one must eat whole foods that contain them. Some vitamins can be absorbed if they are a "food-based formulation" that contains all of the necessary components to absorb the vitamin.
- White table salt. It is toxic, and no one should consume it!
- Anything containing caffeine. Caffeine is bad for multiple organ systems, especially the adrenal glands and the brain. Avoiding caffeine means avoid green tea/herbal teas with caffeine/coffee and more. Do not consume it! Just because something comes from a plant does not mean it's good for you're either. Avoid it at all cost.
- Protein powders. If you want protein, eat a whole food that contains it.
- Factory farmed eggs/meat/fish.
- MSG and food preservatives. If you avoid processed foods entirely, you should be able to avoid these easily.
- Processed lunch meats and heavily processed sausages.
- Drugs and alcohol. They are not ideal substances to have in the human body.

Many people will look at the list of "a bad diet" and think "wow! I cannot eat anything now!" That is far from the truth. There are millions of food choices that do not fit into that category. Most grocery stores are filled with food that is not fit for human consumption. Many people were raised to think that these foods are made for humans, so making changes to most peoples diet, can be as radical as changing their religion. The best way to look at it is to say "what does my body need?"

Do not try to find replacements for foods that you cannot eat. Many people, when told to avoid something, try to find a way around it. If they cannot eat gluten, they find gluten free bread (even though they are unhealthy). If someone wants to avoid meat, they will make "vegan burgers", which are nearly always unhealthy. If you cannot find a healthy alternative, it should not be eaten. I understand that people are used to eating bread/pasta/burgers/pizza, and will try to find alternatives. You can try to do this, but usually it is a lot easier to find new recipes that accommodate a nutritious diet. Raw foodist's and paleo recipe books have plenty of great ideas. I am personally lazy and hate preparing food. Instead of making a salad, I just put the vegetables in my mouth and eat them. It is way faster, and I get the nutrients my body so craves.

The Food List

This food list is not complete, but should give you a basic idea of what to eat. This world is filled with millions of edible plants and animals. You need fresh foods complete with nutrients. Here are some examples:

Vegetables:

- Arugula
- Asparagus
- Avocado
- Beets
- Broccoli
- Capers
- Cauliflower
- Crookneck squash
- Cucumbers
- Fennel bulb
- Horseradish
- Leek
- Lettuce (All Kinds)
- Kale
- Mushrooms
- Mustard greens
- Onions
- Sweet Potatoes or Yams
- Spinach
- Swiss chard
- Watercress
- Yams
- Celery

Sprouts

- Alfalfa
- Broccoli
- Buckwheat
- Mung Bean
- Red clover
- Fenugreek
- Mustard seed
- Wheat Grass
- Sunflower
- Lentils
- Chickpeas
- Almonds

Berries

- Bilberry
- Blackberry
- Boysenberry
- Blueberry
- Cranberry
- Hawthorne Berry
- Juniper Berry
- Loganberry
- Mulberry
- Raspberry
- Red currant
- Strawberry

Fruits

- Apricot
- Cherries
- Coconut
- Figs
- Guava
- Honeydew melon
- Kiwi
- Lemon
- Lime
- Mandarin orange
- Nectarine
- Olives
- Papaya
- Passion fruit
- Peach
- Pear
- Persimmon
- Pineapple
- Plum
- Pomegranate (Raw only, not the juice they sell in stores!)
- Star fruit
- Tangerine

Animal Products (Only 4 Ounces at every meal. Must be organic/wild!)

- Beef/Lamb/Wild Game/Venison/ Poultry/ Organ Meats (especially organic animal livers)
- Organic Pasture Raised Eggs
- Wild Caught Fish and Shellfish that is low in mercury. I find that sardines are the best choice

Natural Sweeteners

- Stevia

Nuts and Seeds (Should be soaked or sprouted before consumption)

- Walnuts
- Almonds
- Sunflower seeds
- Flaxseed
- Pumpkin seeds
- Brazil nuts
- Anise seed
- Pine nuts
- Cashews

Healthy Oils (Must be Extra Virgin/Cold Pressed)

- Avocado Oil
- Apricot Kernel Oil
- Almond Oil
- Flaxseed Oil
- Olive Oil
- Hazelnut Oil

Miscellaneous

- Nutritional Yeast Flakes
- Sauerkraut (Only Raw. Most on the market are not)
- Spirulina
- Pickled Vegetables
- Apple Cider Vinegar
- Fresh/Raw Wheat Grass Juice
- Bone Broths

Methods to solve the pain before having the surgery

Most alternative therapies will not give you results. You might feel a little bit better, but you will find yourself frustrated as the months go by, and you are still in pain.

I have thrown thousands of dollars at Prolotherapy/PRP/Graston and other alternative therapies that help most chronic injuries, but do nothing for a torn labrum. The only therapy that gave me long term pain relief was trigger point therapy, taping and basic physical therapy shoulder stability exercises. Everything you need to know to try these therapies is in the pages of this book. The first thing we need to start with is trigger point therapy.

Keep in mind that the labrum is not causing most of your pain. Trigger points are the biggest culprit. Trigger point work will make the muscles fire properly, causing joint stability. You want to make the shoulder joint as stable as possible before you have surgery, regardless of the pain.

Many physical therapists will tell you to "strengthen the stabilizer muscles" to increase shoulder joint stability. Problem is that a muscle is impossible to strengthen, until the trigger points are resolved. Working out a muscle that has trigger points, will cause more problems. Also, if a muscle has a trigger point, it is inherently weak. Fix the trigger points first, then working on strengthening exercises later on.

Trigger Point Guidelines

Trigger points are tender spots of tissue in the muscle that are made in response to any and all structural injuries in the body. Their purpose is to cause pain when you move a damaged area of the body. This is to force you to rest so that your body can fix the damage in the injury. These trigger points are great for fixing normal injures and forcing someone to rest, but if you have a torn labrum that will never heal without surgery, the trigger points are causing you more harm than good.

The best way to find these trigger points is to carefully massage around the areas I suggest for each muscle and try to find tender areas that hurt to rub. What we want to do is slowly rub each trigger point with blunt force until it is less tender. When it is less tender, or the muscle itself feels softer, then we know we are done. For some muscles, this can be a slow but forceful rub with 6 to 12 slow strokes (a slow and focused massage).

Sometimes rubbing a trigger point will have a "good pain", like when you get knots massaged out of your back. The key to releasing trigger points is to not apply too much pressure. It is best not to go more than 6 out of 10 on the pain scale, where 0 is no pain, and 10 is the most pain.

When we have chronic shoulder pain, and find that trigger point therapy can reduce our pain, some of us will rub the trigger points too hard in a desperate attempt to get rid of the pain. It is much better to keep at 6 out of 10 on the pain scale, and do a lot of consistent small sessions of trigger point work, than it is to do an inconsistent number of "hard" sessions. 3 small sessions a day is much better for you than 1 hard session once a day.

Using tools will allow you to use more pressure on a trigger point than you can with just your hands. I also suggest trying to use tools whenever you can in order to avoid using your thumbs. Thumbs can be damaged by using them too much to rub out trigger points.

Some people will have to hit all the trigger points; some will only have a couple of active trigger points. Sometimes you will not only find a tender spot, but you might find a small nodule or lump or tight band in the muscle as well. This is what a trigger point feels like. You need to slowly massage this out until it is not as tender as when you started. Rubbing them back and forth is the best way to do this. Rub them nice and slowly. If you apply too much pressure to these little trigger points, you will have more pain and more problems. If you massage them nice and softly and have a medium amount of pain while doing so, you will have less pain and fewer problems with your injury. If you do not feel a tender spot, try pushing harder and deeper into the tissues. Sometimes they like to hide pretty deep inside a muscle.

After a few sessions of trigger point therapy, you may feel like your tender spots have become less sensitive and that you might be fine without any more trigger point work. This is wrong. Keep feeling the muscles and search for new trigger points. Sometimes after doing the superficial (surface) layer of muscles, you will later find a whole new set of trigger points deeper in the muscle. These ones will usually require more focused pressure in order to release them. If you do not see results, try pushing a bit harder. Just keep with it daily and do not give up!

You can do these trigger point release methods any time throughout the day. If you are in a lot of pain, doing them 6 times a day is fine (6 light sessions is better than 1 intense session a day). If the area becomes extremely sore or feels more tender, let the area rest and come back to it in a day or two. Your body will adapt to the trigger point therapy quickly, and it is not unusual for you to be able to double the amount of therapy sessions and pressure that you use on the trigger points in as little as 2-3 weeks. It is important to slowly ease into the treatments and to build up to more sessions and more applied pressure while massaging. Listen to your body and respond accordingly.

Trigger Point Tools

It is great to use your hands for diagnostic evaluation of a muscle in question and we will use our hands to deactivate the trigger points, but it is much more ideal to use a trigger point tool when you can. A tool will do quite a few things at once:

- Focus the mechanical pressure to a small area, thus going deeper and also getting hard-to-find trigger points.

- Save our hands from damage. Pressing into trigger points six times a day can beat your hands up pretty quickly and cause more issues. Avoid this at all costs!

- Some tools work well for some muscles, and not so well for others. Use the muscle guides ahead to understand which tools are best suited for releasing certain trigger points.

The following pages contain common trigger point tools that we will use in this book. Most of them are available online and at economical prices.

Lacrosse Ball:

This is my favorite trigger point therapy tool. It is small, light, and effective and can be used on nearly all muscles if you get creative. It is crazy cheap and lasts forever. By the way, do not use a tennis ball; they are HORRIBLE for trigger point massage.

The Back Buddy ©

This tool is nearly required for all labrum injuries. It is one of my favorite tools. It is really useful for self-therapy if you do not have someone around (especially when you must do 6 small trigger point sessions a day). I also find it better than a trigger point therapist in some ways because you can find exact trigger point locations and be able to rub them out accordingly. This tool can help you resolve neck/back pain from your shoulder labrum.

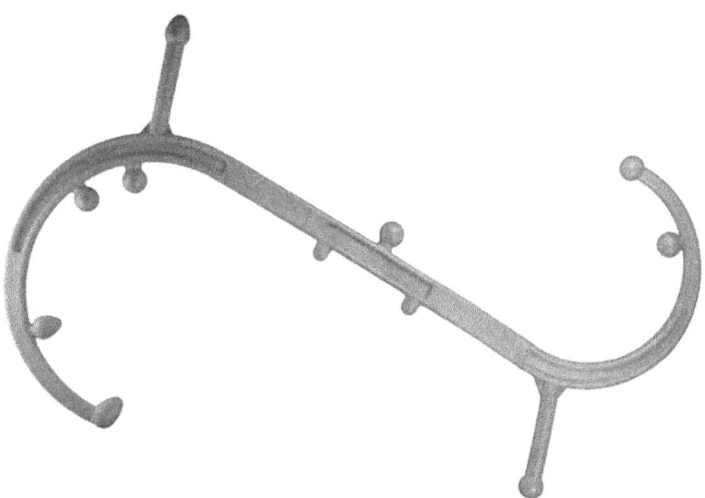

Pros:

- Sturdy, does not flex like other massage sticks even if you are using it to massage really deep.

- Great for places you cannot reach.

- Great assortment of different knobs in very well thought-out places. One side has rounded knobs for a light massage, and the other end has pointy knobs so you can go REALLY deep into the tissues.

Cons:

- It is heavy. If your arms are extremely weak from a recent shoulder injury, it may be hard to use at first.

- Hard to bring with you everywhere you go. I leave mine on the side of my seat in my car so I can always get to it easily.

- Hard to get used to for some. It can take some practice to be able to use it. There are so many ways to use this stick that it is hard to find the ways that best help you at first.

Tip: If you need to massage your back, and you are in your car, put one end of the stick around your back, and the other end of the stick around the steering wheel. This makes it so you can lean your whole weight on the massage stick. I do not suggest using this on small muscles or neck muscles.

Air Hockey Apparatus:

These things are great for back muscles and so much more. Also you can use it in place of a lacrosse ball. This tool will be much more aggressive than a lacrosse ball, but can go deep.

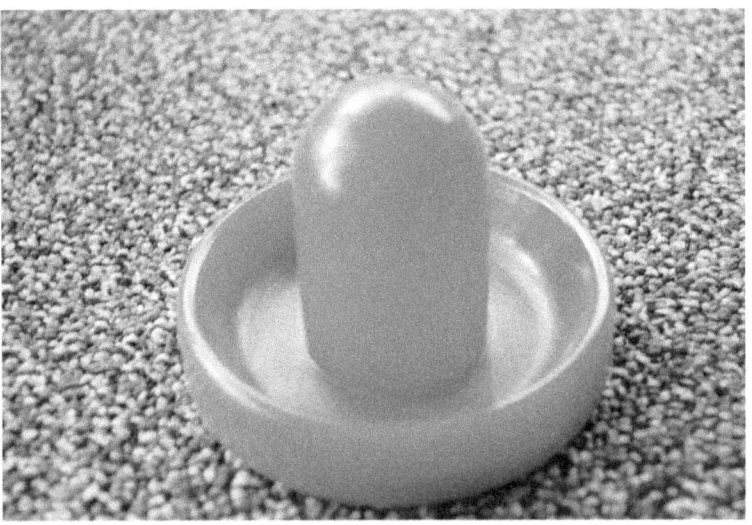

My favorite homemade tool:

Find some sort of rounded peg. Then find a small piece of wood. Drill hole in the wood and put peg into the hole with glue. Now you have one of the best massage tools on the planet! ☺ You can use this for all sorts of trigger points on the body.

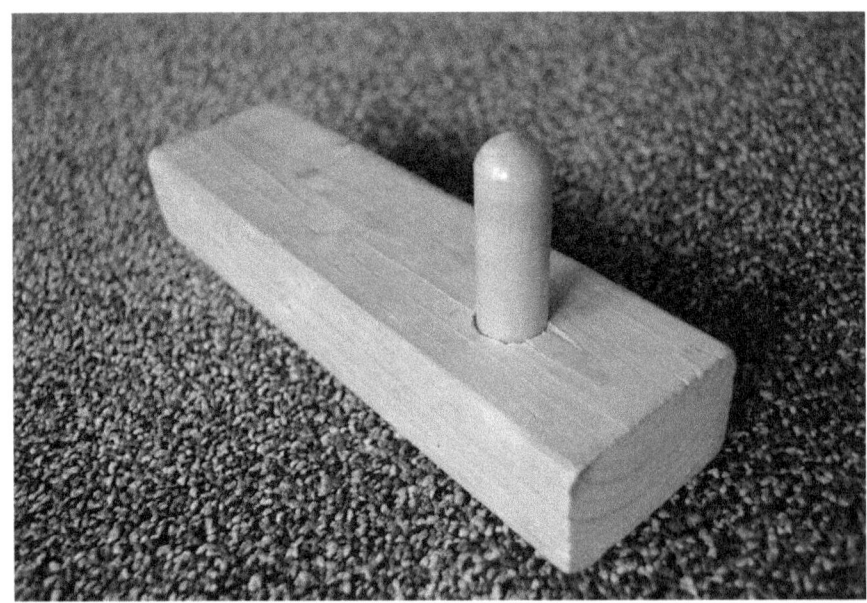

Muscles that we need to treat With Trigger Point Therapy

Muscles to Treat (biggest troublemakers first):

1. Infraspinatus
2. Scalenes
3. Subscapularis
4. Coracobrachialis
5. Supraspinatus
6. Pectoralis Major/Pectoralis Minor
7. Biceps Brachii
8. Trapezius
9. Serratus Anterior
10. Subclavius
11. Levator Scapulae
12. Deltoid

This is a list of the muscles that harbor trigger points that are causing you pain. You want to start at the top of the list, and work through all of the muscles. In the following pages, you will find instructions on how to deal with trigger points for every muscle on this list. You will quickly find that half of the muscles will be ok, and half will be filled with trigger points (for some, all of the muscles will have trigger points).

Once a muscle does not have trigger points, you do not need to treat it for the time being. But keep checking back on all of your muscles because trigger points love to move around because once you fix one area of your shoulder, then other areas like to compensate and can form new trigger points in response.

These trigger points can actually perpetuate the problem as well. If you have a trigger point in the subscapularis, then the humerus can shift anteriorly causing a subluxation, which can tear your labrum even more!

Infraspinatus

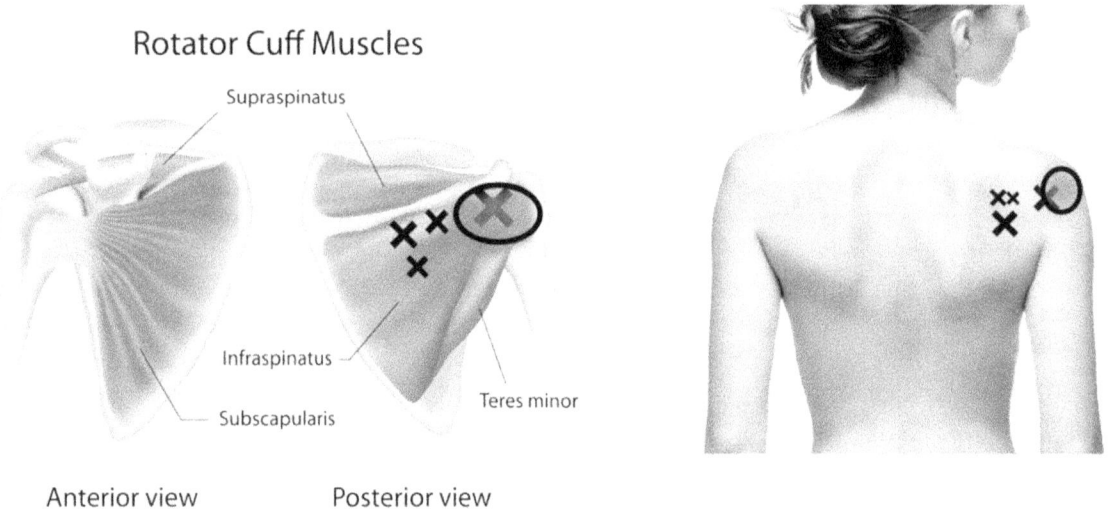

Rotator Cuff Muscles

Supraspinatus

Infraspinatus

Subscapularis

Teres minor

Anterior view   Posterior view

Trigger Point Treatment:

"Back buddy stick" (available on amazon.com) is a great tool to get rid of trigger points in this muscle. Another great tool is a lacrosse ball against a wall. Rub the ball or stick into the "X's" that are depicted in the pictures above. The circle is a common spot for tenderness.

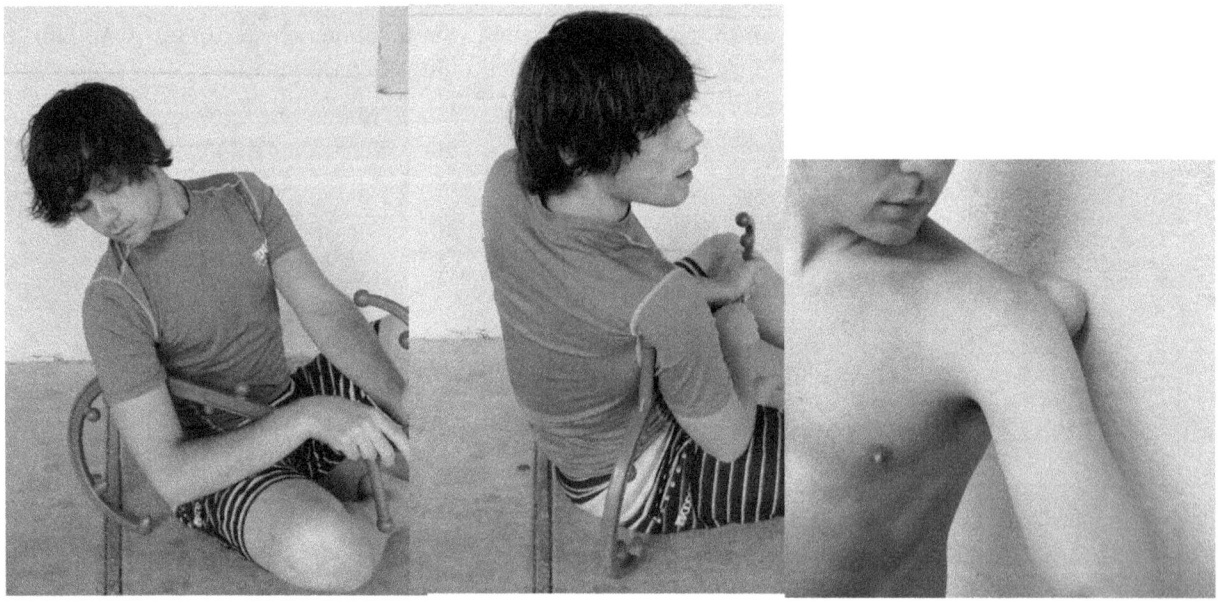

Scalene Group

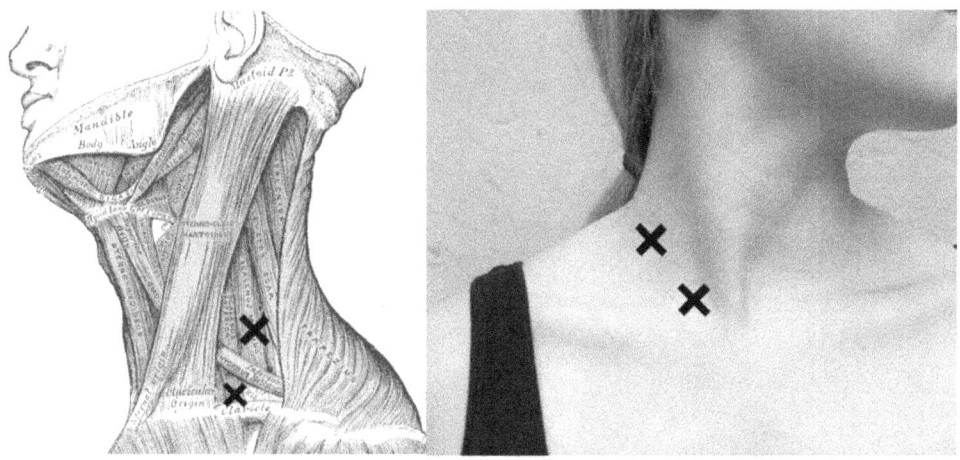

This is a tricky muscle group. It can cause pain far away from the muscle, including the hand and shoulder. I personally had so much pain from this muscle alone after my last shoulder surgery, and if left untreated, can make you have 24/7 pain in your shoulder and hand. Muscle dysfunction can also cause nerve entrapment due to the nerve bundle that passes through this muscle group. This muscle can cause pain to radiate in the front of the shoulder, and commonly has trigger points in everyone with a torn labrum.

Trigger Point Treatment:

What you need to do to get to this muscle is feel for the Sternocleidomastoid muscle. If you turn your head in either direction, you will see a muscle in the front of the neck. It looks like a big rope:

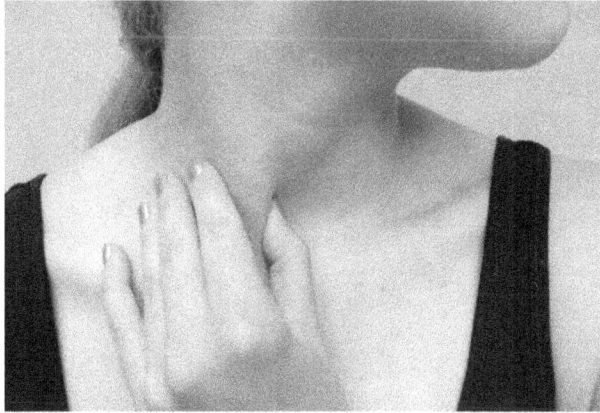

You can grab this muscle and feel that it starts on the chest, and ends on the back of the skull. Once you find this muscle, move it out of the way with your hand (move it towards your throat) and right under this muscle lies the Anterior Scalene. The picture above shows the location of the sternocleidomastoid muscle, and how to grab it.

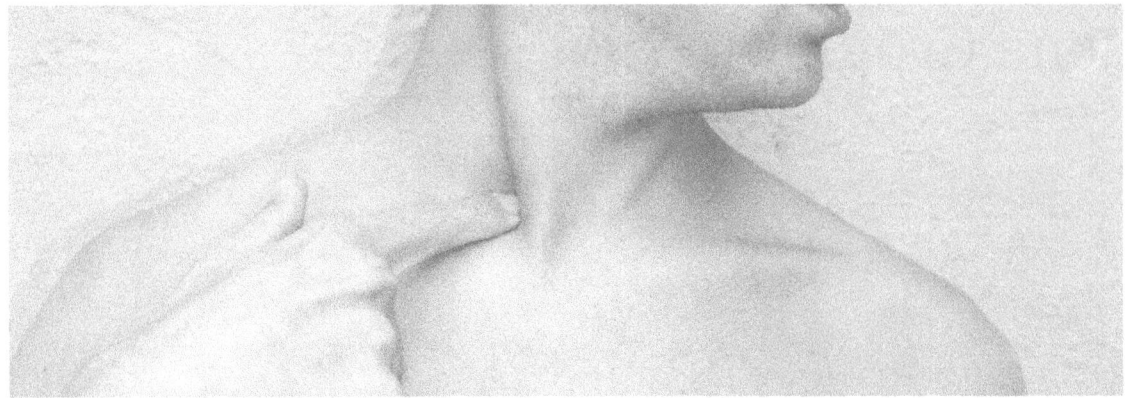

After you move the sternocleidomastoid, you will be able to reach the anterior scalene muscle. The picture above shows where you should massage. It will more than likely be tender.

Slowly massage it out. If you hit a nerve, it will be painful. If you go slowly and carefully, you should not hit any nerves. The nerves feel like ropes next to the muscles. Just feel around for muscle knots and they should be pretty obvious when you hit them. Use your fingers to slowly massage them out.

The Posterior Scalene and Middle Scalene (the "X" in the picture that is closer to your back) can be massaged by having someone push an elbow into this area. You can also massage it yourself with your hands, but it can be very difficult. Watch out for the nerve that passes next to the Middle Scalene muscle. Using a back buddy bar© is a great option as well.

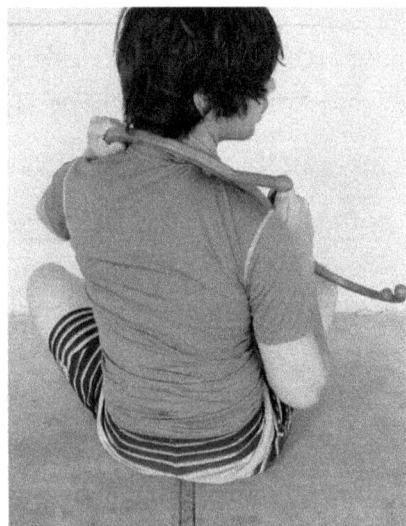

If this is at all confusing to you, check out http://www.mstrtherapy.com for a video on how to treat this muscle. You can find it under the treatment video section under shoulder pain.

Subscapularis

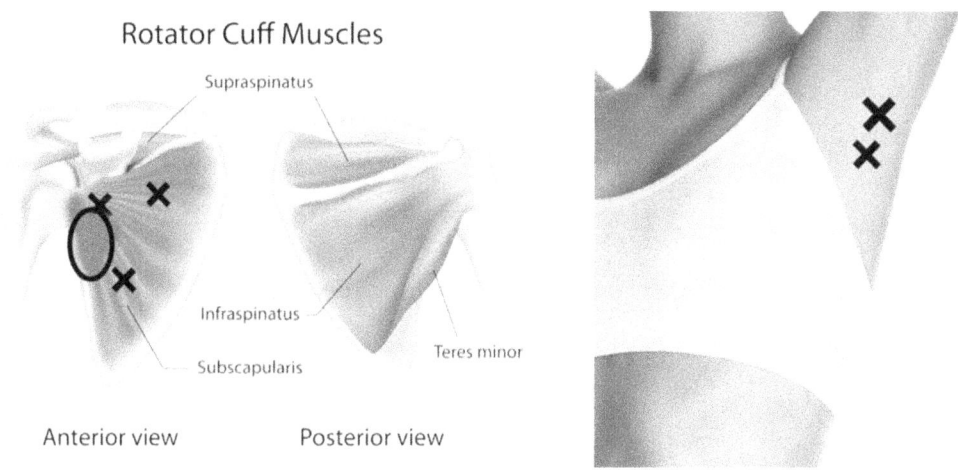

Rotator Cuff Muscles

Supraspinatus

Infraspinatus

Subscapularis

Teres minor

Anterior view   Posterior view

Trigger Point Treatment:

Using various poles, including the small poles with rounded ends on The Back Buddy © stick, works really well to get this muscle working properly again. The trigger points are very near to nerves, so if you feel a pain that is not a trigger point pain, do not push on the area.

This muscle is really hard to massage properly. Just imagine that it is in the back wall of the armpit. It is literally under the scapula (on the front side of the scapula, which moves on the backs rib cage).

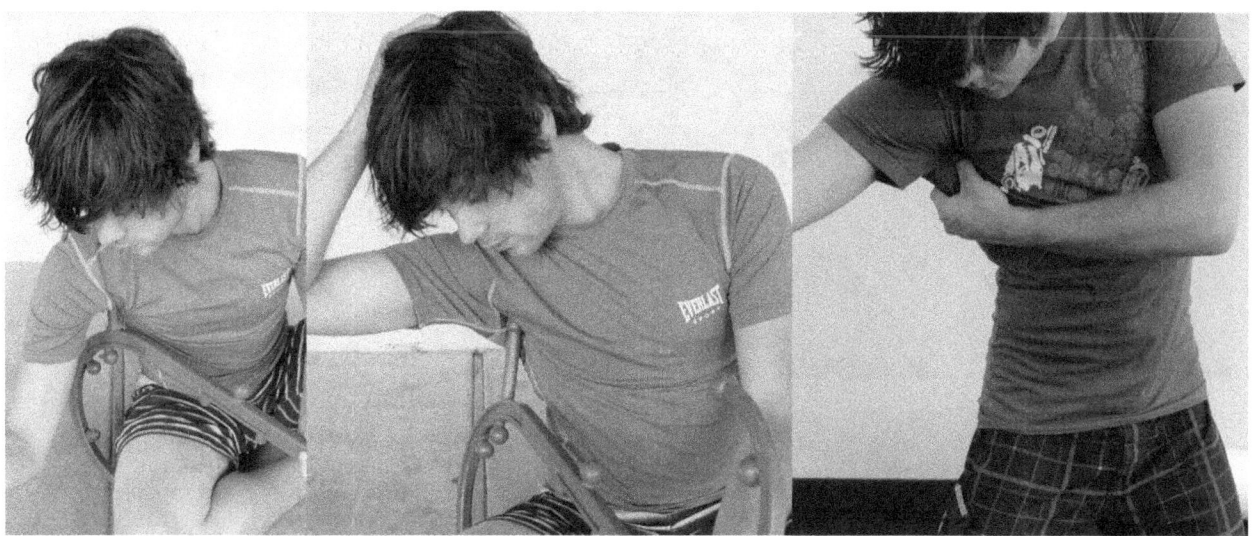

Coracobrachialis

This little muscle loves to cause a ton of pain in the front of the shoulder. It is responsible for raising your arm in front of you (flexion) and also assists in adduction of the shoulder joint. This muscle is hard to find. It lies under the deltoid and is medial (towards the midline of the body) to the biceps brachii.

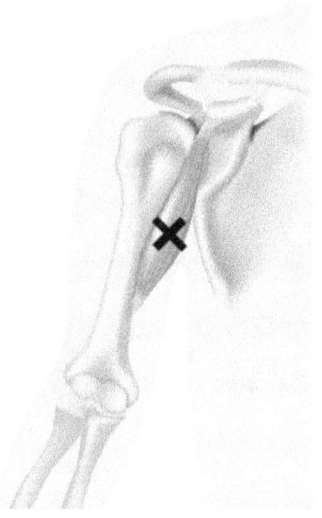 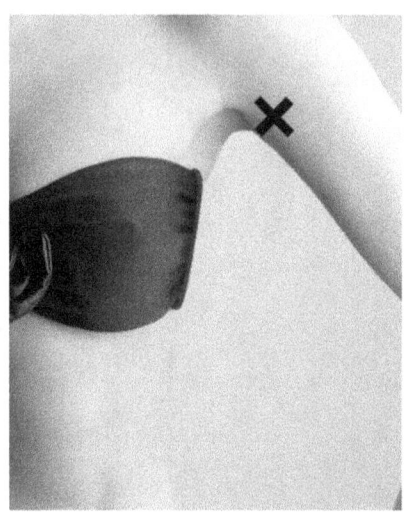

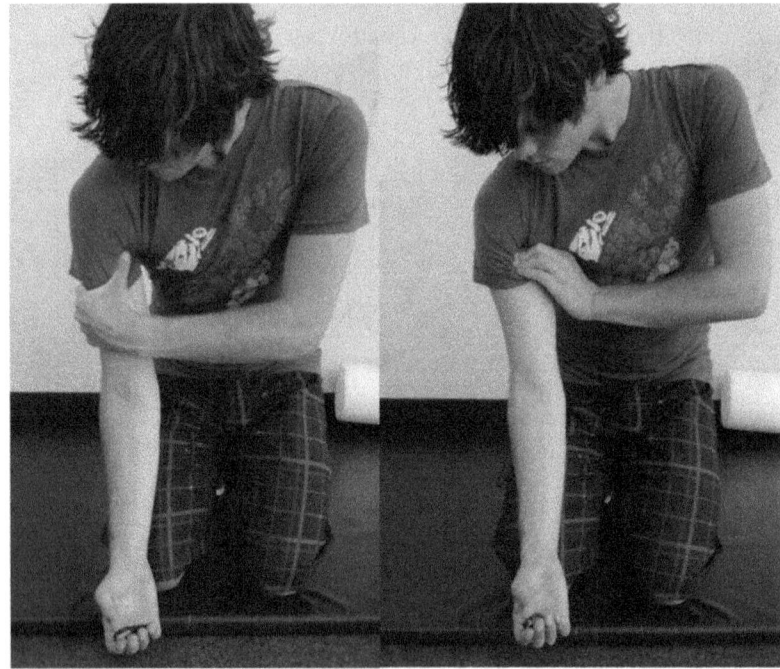

Trigger Point Treatment:

It is hard to find. It is a small muscle and does not require much force to release, so you can safely use your thumb without any problems. The muscle responds well to up and down and side-to-side massage very well. The only issue you may run into is hitting the nerve. There is a nerve that runs just posterior (towards your back) to the coracobrachialis. It will feel very sensitive if you hit it. Just make sure you progress to higher amounts of pressure slowly. You should be looking for a "tender point" that feels good to massage. If you hit an area that is tender, but does not feel like the usual "feel good muscle massage" feeling, than you are on a nerve. Take a good look at the photo above to figure out the location of this muscle.

Supraspinatus

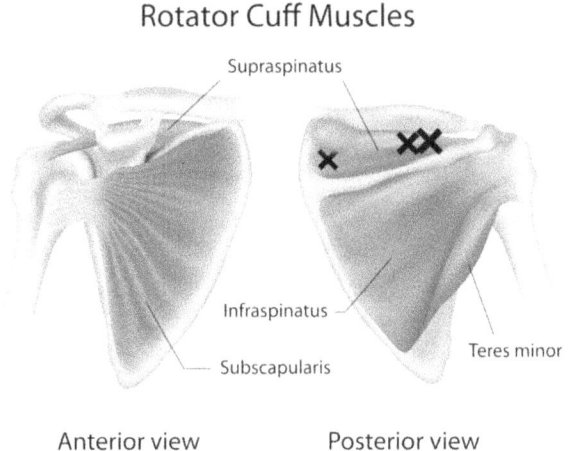

Rotator Cuff Muscles

Supraspinatus

Infraspinatus

Subscapularis

Teres minor

Anterior view   Posterior view

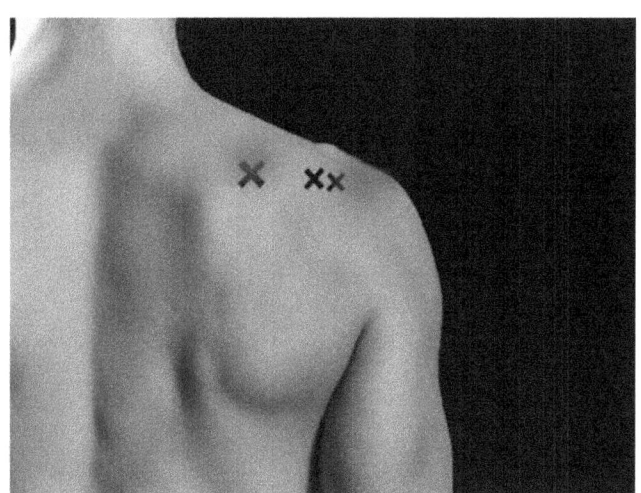

Trigger Point Treatment:

This muscle is hard to treat properly. This muscle is somewhat deep and lies under the Trapezius. In order to treat, just push straight into it. I find that it helps to have someone dig their elbow into this muscle while you are lying down. If you can't find someone to do that, use a back buddy stick. Lacrosse balls work for some people. I suggest trying to get someone to dig their elbow in more than anything because it is so effective.

Use the spine of the scapula to reference (long bony bump that goes across your scapula and goes toward your shoulder joint) and massage right above it. There is a little canyon just above the spine of the scapula and this is where the Supraspinatus is.

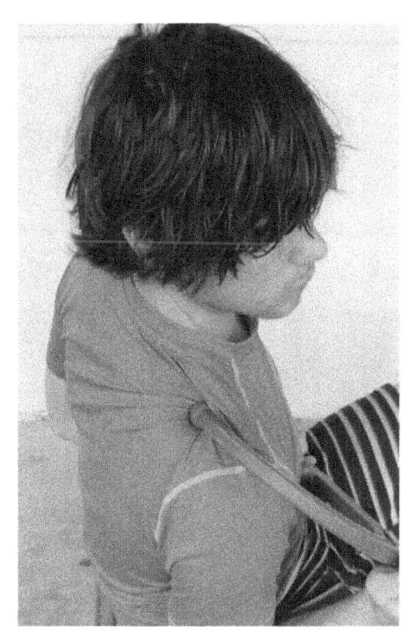

Pectoralis Major

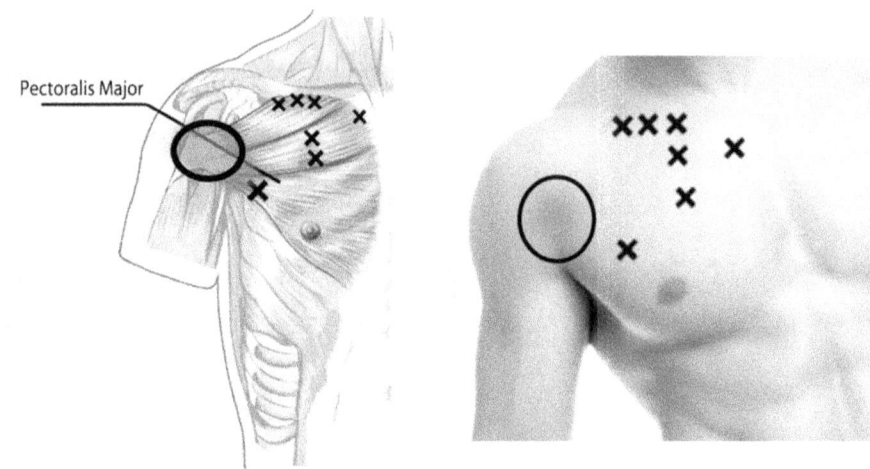

Trigger Point Treatment:

Use a lacrosse ball against a wall. Most important thing to do here is to check every part of the muscle. There are fibers that extend up to the clavicle and sternum. You must check every area out. Press the lacrosse ball into the circle area for an extended amount of time. Should feel a little tender at first.

Pectoralis Minor

This is a very important muscle for scapular stability. If you are in a desk hunched over a computer all day, this muscle will be shortened and tender. Luckily, it is easy to treat and responds well to trigger point treatment.

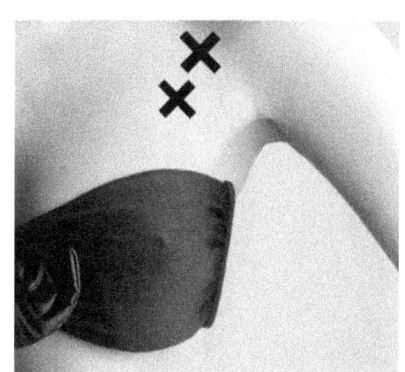

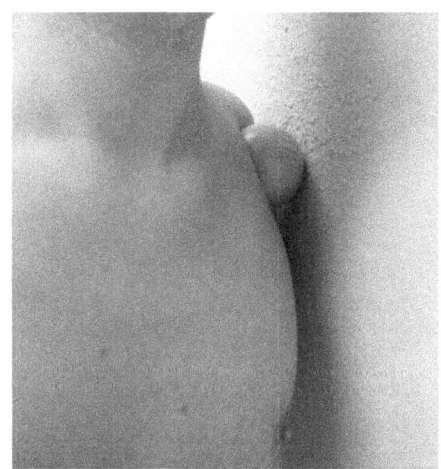

Trigger Point Treatment:

Use a lacrosse ball against a wall to treat this muscle's trigger points. In order to get deep into the muscle, move your shoulder forward and backward (protraction/retraction) while pushing the lacrosse ball into the muscle. This will make the treatment much more effective.

Biceps Brachii

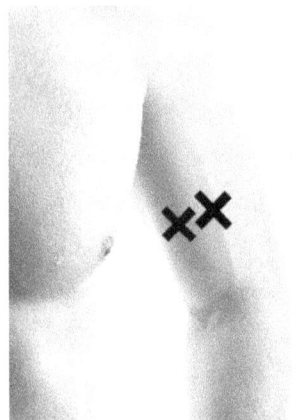

It is really common for this muscle to become dysfunctional and cause elbow and shoulder pain. It is overworked in lots of athletes which lead to muscle imbalances. The long head of this muscle travels in a small sheath near the shoulder and attaches to the scapula. This area is prone to injury and ruptures to these muscles tendons are not uncommon.

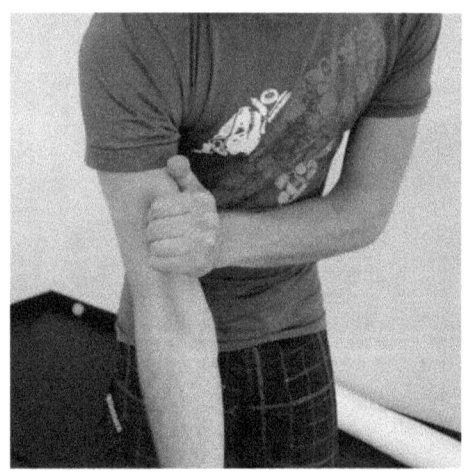

Trigger Point Treatment:

Every area of this muscle is easy to palpate, so trigger point therapy is pretty easily done. You can usually use your hands for the treatments if you do not use your thumbs (grab the muscle with the fingers). It is easy to find tender points in this muscle, and they can respond pretty quickly to treatment.

Trapezius

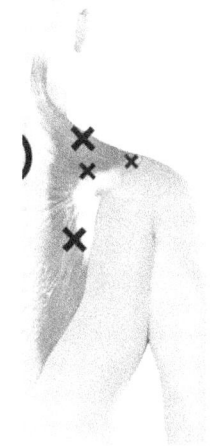 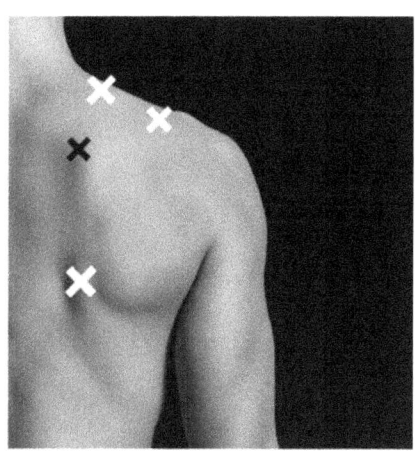

This muscle commonly feels good to massage. The reason is because it loves to become dysfunctional in the office worker. If you have to hunch over a desk all day, this muscle will be chronically lengthened and full of trigger points. Another implication to take into consideration is the fact that the Trapezius muscle deals with multiple angles of force. Some parts of the muscle make the scapula move one direction; others make the scapula move in the opposite direction. This can make the Trapezius's job extremely demanding and make it vulnerable to dysfunction. If the muscle is used frequently in someone with good posture and an active lifestyle, it is very hard for it to become dysfunctional. The instant you sit at a desk, and hunch over a keyboard, this muscle get put in a position that it should not be in. If this muscle has been bothering you for months on end and the trigger points do not seem to want to go away, try to release the Serratus Anterior and Pectoralis Minor. If that helps, also try doing shoulder rolls and shrugs every hour or so to get the muscle back into shape. Technically, it will not be technically "stronger", but more articulate with its movements (fine tuning your neurofacilitation mechanisms).

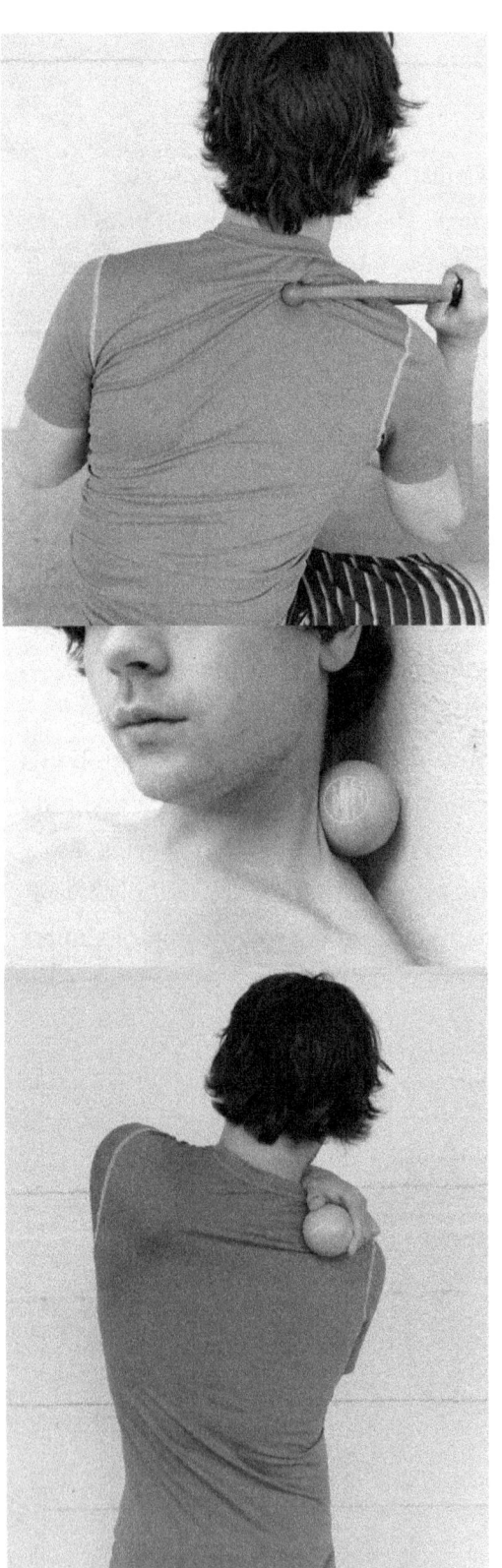

Trigger Point Treatment:

There are many trigger point treatment options. Use a Lacrosse ball against a wall. Also use a foam roller across the upper back. Back buddy stick can work as well for some of the big trigger points.

Serratus Anterior

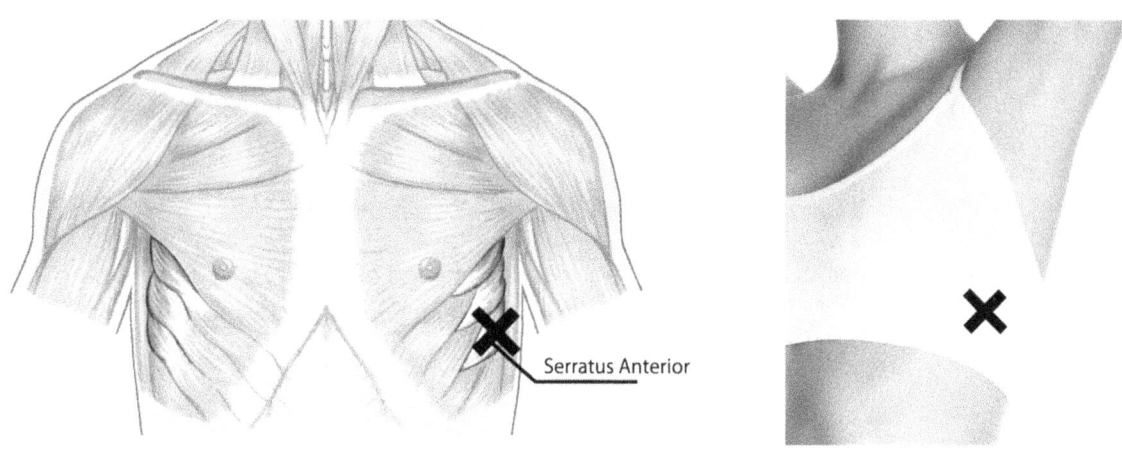

Serratus Anterior

This is an important scapula stabilizer and also assists in breathing. When this muscle is dysfunctional, it can hurt to breathe. If you have to expel air out of the lungs fast, such as sneezing or coughing, this muscle will shoot pain all over your sides and mid back. It is responsible for protracting your scapula and in most people it will be inhibited or weak.

Trigger Point Treatment:

Wrap your arm around your side and feel this muscles location for its main trigger point. It may take a second of feeling around, but when you find this trigger point, you will know it. It is usually pretty sensitive and feels really good to massage out.

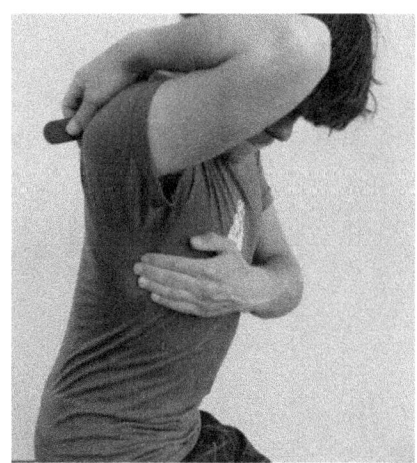

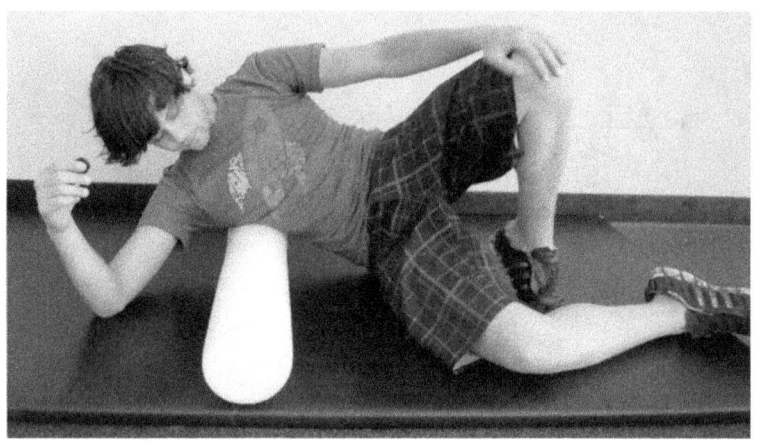

You can also lie on a foam roller and massage this area out. Should be a big foam roller and you should not over arch your back when you lay on it.

Subclavius

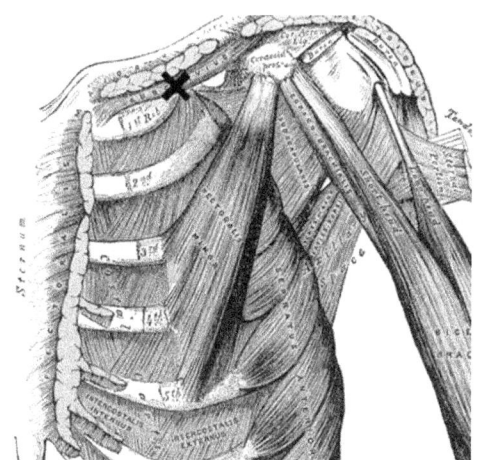

This is a small muscle, but it can cause a lot of pain. Luckily, it is easy to treat.

Trigger Point Treatment:

Simply use a lacrosse ball against a wall. Lift up your shoulder and push the ball under your Clavicle (collarbone). Slowly push the ball into the muscle and let your shoulder hang down. Relax and push the ball into the trigger points.

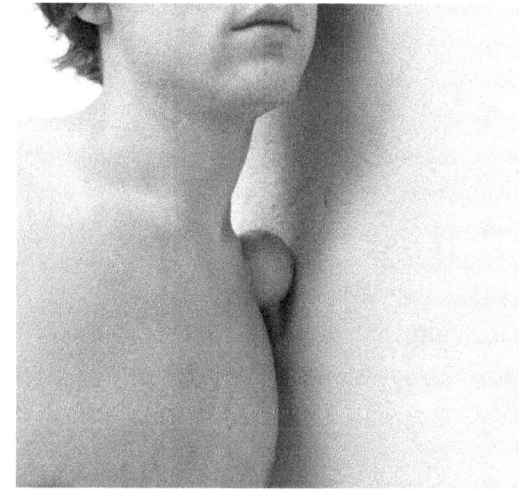

Levator Scapulae

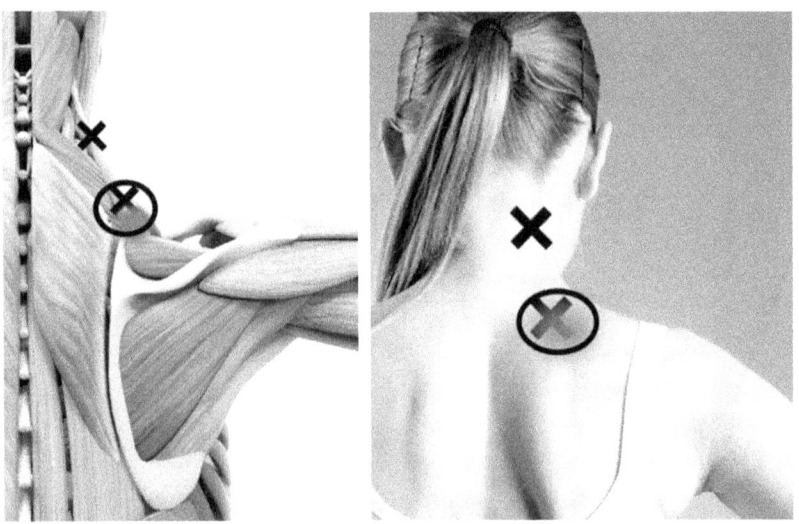

Trigger Point Treatment:

Rub this thing out with a back buddy stick© or with lacrosse ball against a wall. It feels really good to rub this muscle out.

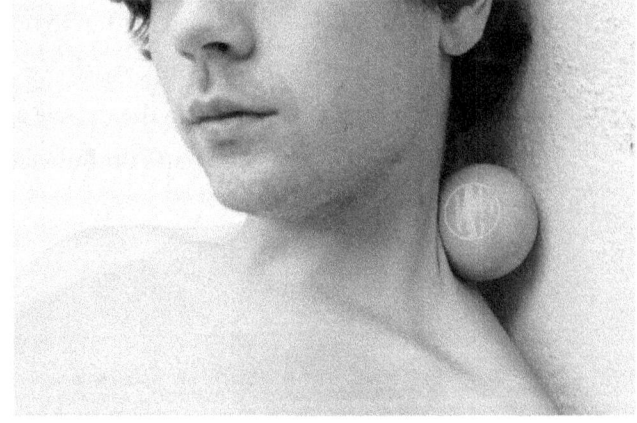

Deltoid

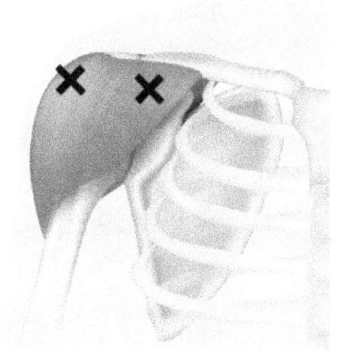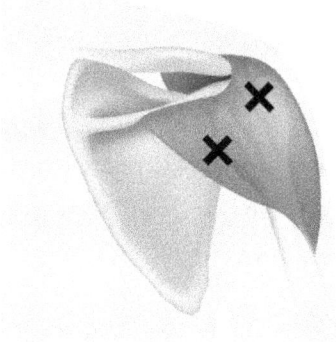

Anterior view   Posterior view

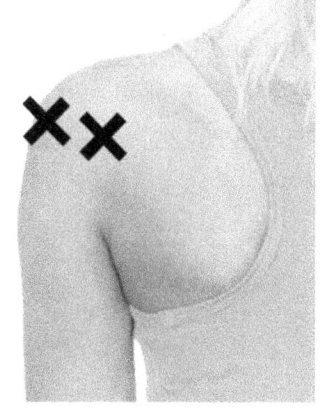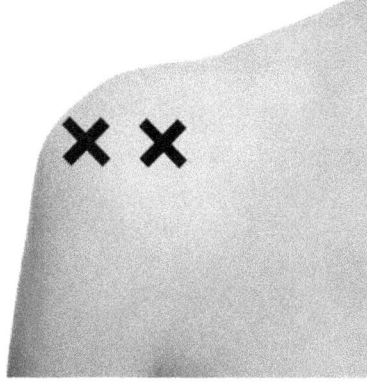

This is a multi-articulate muscle with a wide variety of movements. Muscle fiber in the deltoid start and end in various areas, and the muscle is extremely important for shoulder stability. Because the shoulder is very prone to instability issues, this muscle needs to be functioning properly to stabilize the shoulder joint.

Usually this muscle is not dysfunctional on its own, and dysfunction in this muscle is more of a side effect of having dysfunction in other muscles, such as the Pectoralis Major, Scalene muscles, and Rotator Cuff muscles.

Trigger Point Treatment:
The best way to treat all the trigger points of this muscle is without a doubt by using a lacrosse ball against a wall.

Taping a Labrum Tear

Taping can help a great many of you, but not all. Also, taping is a skill that requires practice. Sometimes you will tape, and it will cause more pain. Do not become discouraged. Instead you need to try different taping methods till you find one that works for you.

Most taping methods for a torn labrum have to do with stability. The tape will keep the shoulder in a healthy range of motion so that it does not tear further. There are many different ways to tape a shoulder for all around stability, and a simple youtube video search will show you many various methods. Kinesiotape (elastic athletic tape) is a great option as well.

Before you tape, you must wash your shoulder with bar soap and water. Do not use lotion soaps or hand sanitizer. You need the basic white bar soap. Use the soap to clean off the shoulder, in a shower, and then pat it down till its dry. Do not try to tape without doing this! The tape will fall off if the skin is not completely clean and free of oils.

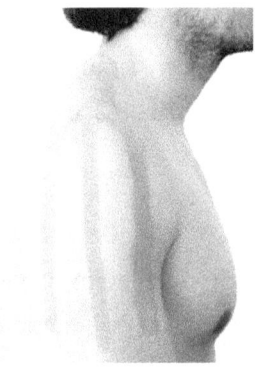

In this picture we see a basic tape job for shoulder stability. This one should give most people decent results. If you use thick athletic tape strips, such as white/leukotape, use separate pieces of tape to replace the pieces that are going down the front and side of the shoulder.

If you have scapular stability issues, which can happen from muscle imbalances, this taping job may help you. I like to extend the top piece of tape down to the front of the shoulder.

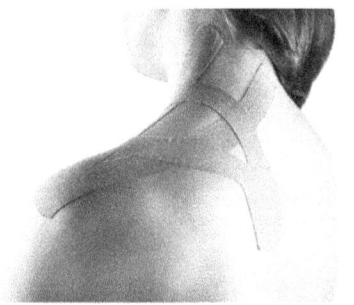

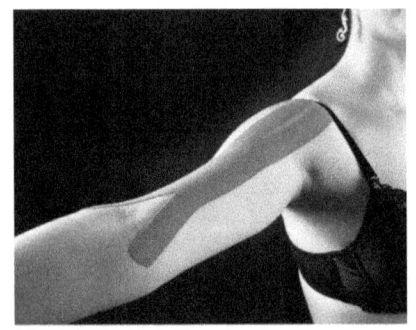

If you have a classic SLAP tear with biceps involvement, this taping job may help you. This is my personal favorite for my labrum tears, but it might not work for everyone. You just have to try it out and see how it feels.

Stability Exercises

After a few weeks of trigger point therapy, your shoulder should feel less pain. If not, work on the trigger points and try to look around for more trigger points that you may have missed.

Strengthening the rotator cuff is the most typical method to promote joint stability in the shoulder. This means that you will have a few exercises that you do 1-2 times a day. They are meant to be done nice and easy, and without a lot of weight. Keep in mind that a stable joint is a strong joint. Focus on promoting strength through joint stability. You do not want to use excessive resistance or weight with these exercises. Over time, and using pain as your guide, you can increase resistance. Let this be a slow process.

Shoulder Joint Stability Movements:

- External Rotation
- Internal Rotation
- Abduction
- Horizontal Abduction
- Flexion

Scapula Stability Movements:

- Retraction
- Elevation

Neck Stability Movements:

- All Around Stability Exercise

Shoulder Stability Movements Guide:

You need to buy an elastic band with the lowest amount of resistance you can find. Do around 20-30 reps of each exercise below. Keep in mind that you want to start off with minimal resistance at first, and increase resistance slowly. If you are in a lot of pain, be careful.

External Rotation:

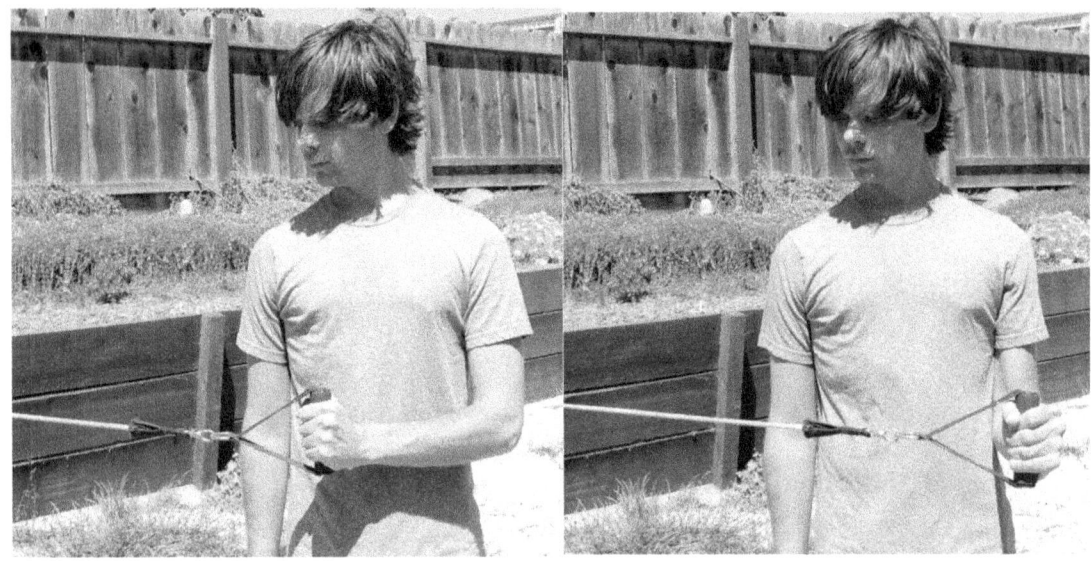

Internal Rotation:

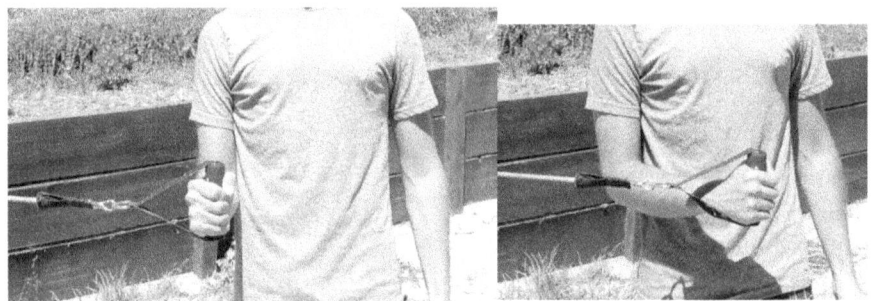

Abduction:

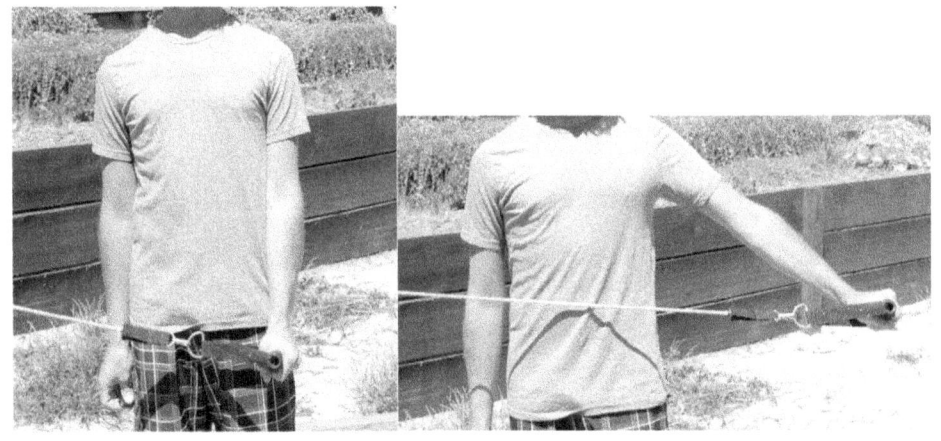

Horizontal Abduction:

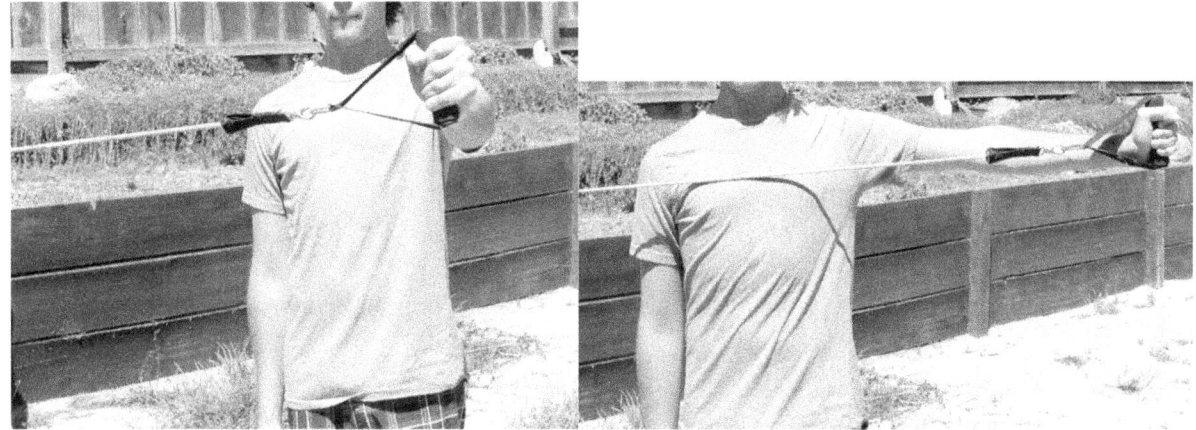

Flexion:

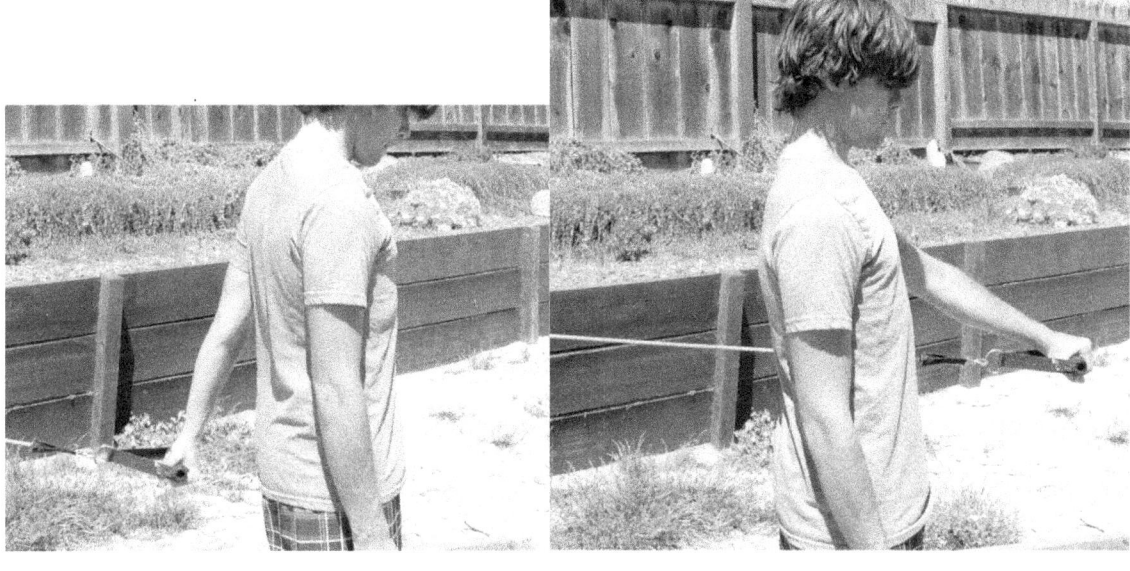

Scapular Stability Movements Guide:

You do not necessarily need to make these muscles "strong" for now. What we want to do is get them moving, and firing properly. Our main goal is joint stability for functionality, then strength later. So do these exercises whenever you are driving/working at a desk/walking around etc. Just squeeze your shoulder blades together and repeat till you feel a nice burn.

For Scapular elevation, just raise your shoulders up to your neck. Commonly referred to as "shoulder shrugs".

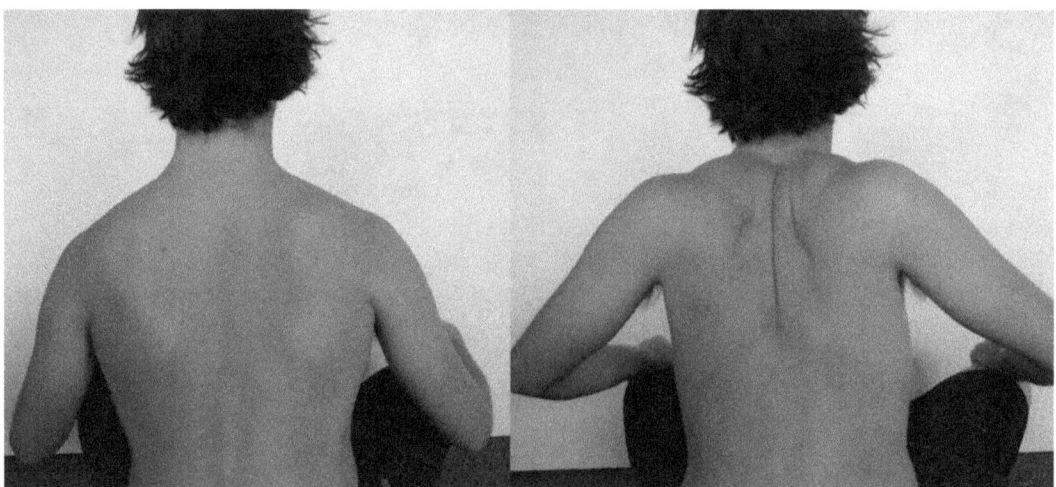

All-Around Neck Stability Exercise

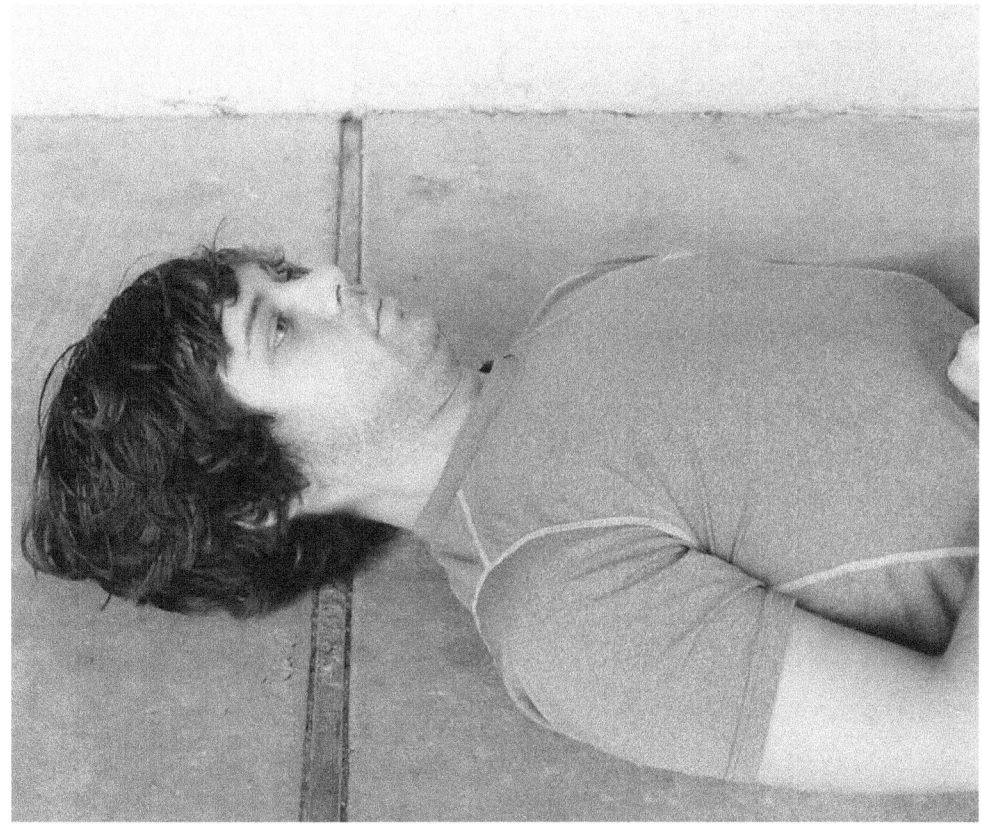

Lie on your back and lift your head a couple centimeters off the ground while making a double chin. This will strengthen the weak muscles in the front of your neck. Make sure you make a slight double chin. Hold the position for 30-60 seconds; less if it is difficult, more if it is easy.

Labrum Repair Surgery

As the years go by, and the pain persists, you will want the surgery. No one likes having shoulder surgeries because it takes at least 4 months to recover from it. This can mean time off work because the first 4-6 weeks, you will be unable to drive. If you have a desk job, you should be ok. If you have a hard labor job, you will need to take at least 5 months off. This is hard to accomplish for most people that need to work to feed their families. If you want the surgery and need to still work, I suggest finding a temporary occupation that you can continue even after you have the surgery.

Keep in mind that the success of the surgery is not determined by the skill of the surgeon, but is also determined by your diet, and how much you move. If you lie in bed all day, and eat a ton of junk food, your surgery will take forever to heal.

When I had my first labrum surgery, it took me 5 months till I could drive again. This is because I also had a nerve disease and I could not walk around much. This slowed down my recovery dramatically. Right now I am recovering from my most recent labrum surgery as I write this book, and at 6 weeks, I am already driving! The reason I healed up so fast is because I resolved my nerve disease and I can walk around. I also can afford supplements that speed up the recovery dramatically.

Make sure that you have some money saved up before you have the surgery, and you have a safe environment to recover in. Finding an insurance company that can pay for the surgery is most ideal, because the cost of the surgery can be quite high. If you are low income, go to a county hospital and see if they have a "low income insurance option". These programs can pay for the entire cost of the surgery if you qualify.

You will want to stockpile some food and supplements before the surgery, and prepare your house for life with "one arm". Also, look for some other options for shoulder slings. The sling that they send you home with after the surgery may be very uncomfortable, and can usually wreak havoc on your posture, causing your neck and back to ache for weeks. Shoulder slings put your arms and neck into an unnatural position, and you need to keep this in mind. Do not let the shoulder sling allow you to slump forward. A lot of people have issues when they come out of the sling due to this bad posture. It also will slow down recovery dramatically, and promote long term pain.

Shoulder Surgery Checklist:

- Safe environment
- Transportation option (no driving permitted for 4-6 weeks)
- Money saved up and a stockpile of food
- Supplements
- Alternative Slings that are more comfortable. Search Amazon.com for double strap slings and other options.
- Temporary Occupation to make money while you recover
- A good insurance plan that will pay for the surgery
- At month 2 (post-surgery), buy a gym pass that gives you access to a pool
- If you can afford it, buy an exercise bicycle for your house. Being able to work out will speed up recovery and prevent boredom
- Time killing activities. I suggest buying some books or start a project you have always wanted to do. I personally read Wikipedia articles and watched documentaries☺. Video games are always a great option as well.
- Have a good source of water for after the surgery. You do not want to depend on tap water. It is poison. Buy a quality filter system. Having clean water can speed up recovery.
- Find a physical therapy clinic that you can travel to by bus or walking. Physical therapy may be started at 4-6 weeks depending on what the surgeon says.
- Try to find a shoulder surgeon. Make sure that whatever surgeon you have; they are comfortable with doing labrum repairs. Shoulder specialists are ideal.
- If you are overweight, you should fix that problem before having the surgery done. Obesity makes everything difficult. Stop eating as much and change your dict now.

How to speed up recovery after the surgery:

- Walk as much as possible! If you sit around all day, it will heal very slowly. Do not stop moving!

- Avoid NSAID's/pain pills after surgery. Some of you may think that this is crazy, but the pain is not that bad. You will have quite a bit of pain when the nerve block wears off, but most people can handle it. NSAID's and pain pills slow down recovery in many ways. Avoid them if you can.

- Ice does not help anything except for pain. It is better to focus on lymphatic drainage (water intake and keeping active) to support the inflammatory response, instead of trying to inhibit it. Inflammation is good, and required for healing. Ice and anti-inflammatory drugs stop the healing process. Focus on having a perfect diet and lots of water.

- After about 4-8 days of wearing the sling, take the sling off while you are sitting down. This will be scary and uncomfortable, but it is good to take it off and relax. I personally find that taking the sling off whenever I am not walking is ideal. The sling can cause more issues than it solves in some instances.

- Keep the arm moving. After 4 days in the sling, move your arm, without actually moving it. Do micro movements while you are in the sling, so that the muscles keep firing. This does not mean working it out, or moving excessively. You want to do these "micro movements" all day. An arm that does small movements will heal much faster than one that hangs in the sling doing nothing.

- If you have a good diet and are walking quite a bit, you should be able to take your sling off early. When my doctor says 6 weeks in the sling, I am out by the 4th week. If the doctor says 4 weeks, such as my most recent surgery, I am out of the sling by 2.5 week. Keep in mind that those suggested recovery times they recommend are for "most people" that are very unhealthy. Stay active and eat a perfect diet, and you will be out of that sling before you know it! If you are unhealthy, and have ANY underlying disorders/diseases, stay in the sling for longer.

- Find an exercise bike if you can. Working out every day will speed up the recovery dramatically. Increasing circulation and promoting growth hormones from working out helps everything.

- Have plenty of sunshine exposure. Vitamin D from the sun will help your bone anchors heal into your scapula. Also make sure your environment is warm. Putting sweaters/jackets on, while in the sling, is very hard to do. It is better to have the surgery during the summer so you can stay in a t-shirt for the first week or so. Dressing can be pretty tough to do with one arm.

- Find food options that are easy to eat. Cooking elaborate and complex recipes will not be possible with one arm. Find health food options that you do not have to prepare. I prefer canned sardines and fresh raw vegetables.

Required Supplements to speed up recovery:

- Trace Minerals and Liquid Magnesium
- Raw Foods Based Calcium Supplement
- Vitamin K2: Mk7 form
- Cod Liver Oil
- Sunshine exposure for Vitamin D synthesis

Not required, but can help speed up recovery and more:

- Systemic Enzymes such as Wobenzym©, Serrapeptase, Bromelain
- Soil Based Organism Probiotics
- Co-Enzyme B-Vitamin
- Buffered Vitamin C
- Milk thistle to expel/detox drugs and toxins used for surgery
- And do not forget: Clean water!!

Keep in mind that after the shoulder surgery, and while the labrum is healing itself to back onto the bone, detrimental effects of immobilization will be setting in. When you do not move a body part, it starts to die. The muscles accommodate for the inactivity by eating the muscles, and circulation decreases. The muscles adapt to the inactivity quickly. Over time, the connective tissue around the muscles accommodates to the static position that the sling forces your arm to be in. Your body "locks up" your arm. This is why it hurts badly to get out of the sling. The body can take a long time to fix the damage dealt to your arm by being stuck in a sling. Your posture will be messed up, and your muscles will be weak. This is why it is so important to keep the arm moving (without moving it. Micro movements are ideal for this purpose). You need to focus on tensing the muscles, without actually moving the shoulder. This does not mean using strength. It means that you should try to contract the muscles lightly. Do some internal/external rotation, flexion and extension, without moving your arm. You can do this in the sling.

Remember that the recovery needs to be very progressive. When you are in the sling, it means that you should be in the sling 24/7 for the first four days, and then by week 2 you should be taking it off at random points of the day so the shoulder does not "freeze up" on you. And by the time you are allowed to take the sling completely off, your arm will already be accustomed to being out of the sling. You want all of the steps to be small, but slowly progressive, day by day.

The first time I had a shoulder labrum surgery, I focused on not moving my arm so that it could heal faster. I figured "keep my arm super still, and once I take off the sling, it will be good to go". I wore the sling 24/7 for 6 weeks without taking it off. I skipped on showers and gave it complete rest. When I came out of the sling, I had issues. My arm was extremely skinny and weaker than it has to be, and it hurt. The pain did not subside for a while. I actually had to still wear the sling for an additional 2 weeks, on and off, just so that I could build up enough strength to take off the sling! I was in pain just to keep my arm dangling by my side. Do not make this mistake!

When you keep a limb motionless in a sling, it slows down healing. When you are in a sling, you need to keep moving. You need to walk around as much as you can, and never stop. This is important because it increases circulation to the area. Even the act of walking will subtly bounce the arm around so that it is getting some sort of motion. When tissues are moving, nutrients are going in, and waste products are going out. Keep on moving! And try to progressively get out of the sling early. Never progress too quickly, or try something out of desperation. You have once chance to get it right.

Trigger Point Therapy after the Surgery

Trigger point therapy is going to be an important tool after the surgery. When you have your arm in a sling for a prolonged amount of time, trigger points will develop. These trigger points are horrid. They are extremely tender, and can cause a lot of pain. Especially from 4 weeks to 10 weeks, you will be dealing with an excessive amount of pain from trigger points. Get that lacrosse ball out and start rubbing various muscles against the lacrosse ball. At week 2-3 after surgery, you should be able to take your sling off and lightly rub the ball against your chest and infraspinatus. Your back may also harbor trigger points, especially in your trapezius muscle, because of the position the shoulder sling puts you in.

When you are in the sling, be sure to keep your posture upright with your shoulders positioned down and back. Try to pinch your shoulder blades lightly (not so much as to damage the shoulder surgery). If you are sitting down all day in your sling, and you slouch your shoulders and extend your neck forward, you will develop trigger points all over your back and neck. This is not fun! Avoid this at all cost.

Over time you will be able to start working out the trigger points in more and more muscles. About an hour before your prescribed physical therapy, work on trigger points. If you have a SLAP tear in the anterior portion of labrum, your subscapularis will be filled with trigger points. This is because they keep your shoulder internally rotate to protect the labrum, so it can heal. If you have a posterior labral tear, than your infraspinatus will be filled with trigger points. Feel around with the lacrosse ball and deal with any trigger points you find. Do not press into them very hard. Trigger points that arise from inactivity are only solved by moving the joint (which you can't do till you are out of the sling), and trigger point therapy. Keep massaging the muscles after the surgery and during the long term recovery. This will speed up muscle firing ability and cause you to heal quickly.

Also, keep looking for trigger points that develop! Just because you get rid of all the trigger points, does not mean that further down the recovery process, trigger points will not develop anymore. Trigger points can come about from the recovery process for the surgery, and from the recovery from having your arm in a compromised and static position (while it was in the sling). You need to fix the trigger points that develop during the entire healing process. Even when you fix all the trigger points, you should feel the areas out with a lacrosse ball once a week.

Physical Therapy Tips for After the Surgery

- Do not progress too quickly. Everything should be a slow and gradual progression, without sudden stressors (working out the shoulder too soon). You can have a fast recovery, if you do everything in a progressive way. Doing physical therapy 3 times a day is ideal, instead of one huge session of physical therapy a day. While writing this I am at 6 weeks post-surgery and I continuously do exercises... all day long. But this does not mean "working hard" at them. I just keep the joint mobile, and the muscles firing. Because I do the exercises all day, the intensity is lower.

- Keep in mind that you are not "strengthening" the muscles when you do physical therapy after the surgery. You are actually re-establishing nerve firing patterns. Your shoulder is atrophied and is not used to moving (from being in the sling). Do not "push it" too early because it can only hurt you.

- Drink plenty of water and take trace minerals. Magnesium is especially helpful because a lot of your muscles will be in a spasm.

- Keep walking! A huge goal that you should have when coming out of the sling is to be able to walk with your arm swinging by your side with your shoulders back. This can take a few weeks to accomplish after coming out of the sling, but this is a great place to be. Having the ability to swing the arms while walking will get the shoulder moving, which will speed up healing. Do not try to swing your arms excessively. Let it happen naturally.

- You will have pain after each session of physical therapy. The pain will last for 20-30 minutes and should be gone after resting the arm. If it stays around for more than 2 hours, and is still sore when you have to do your next physical therapy session, then skip the physical therapy session. Sometimes you will push it too far and you will need to rest it for a day or so. Go by how it feels and do not push through the pain from desperation. Keep in mind that during the exercises, it will hurt a bit. This is fine and normal, but pain that stays around after 2 hours usually means that it needs some rest.

- Alternating between trigger point therapy and exercises is most ideal. The infraspinatus and subscapularis will harbor lots of trigger points when you get out of the sling. Keep massaging these ones LIGHTLY throughout the day with a lacrosse ball. Do not press into these trigger points too hard.

- If you want some guides to the various labrum repair physical therapy exercises, Google search: "Labrum Repair Protocol PDF". You will now have access to thousands of different orthopedic doctor's recommendations on exercises and recovery time suggestions. This is a very useful tool because each doctor will have different recommended times of recovery. Some say that you can drive at 4 weeks, and a few others will say 6 weeks. If you feel that your doctor is wrong about anything, and you feel like he is pushing you too fast, or too slow, check out these recovery protocols. Keep in mind that the more work you have done to your shoulder, the slower they want the recovery process to precede. If you had a small repair, they will want you out of the sling quickly. Some doctors will suggest you to be in the sling for an excessive amount of time, especially if shoulder surgeries are not their specialty. I would ask a physical therapist or other doctor if one is available, to see what their opinion is. If you have bone anchors, 4 weeks will be a typical amount of time in the sling. If you are young and extremely healthy (perfect diet) then 3 weeks is do-able.
- While you are recovering your shoulder, think about the rest of your body. Is your neck hurting from the sling? Is your posture off? Try to correct all of these things so they do not linger about and cause more issues. Check out my website for free treatments for other areas of the body: http://www.mstrtherapy.com
- When you have a full range of motion, but everything is weak, then get into the pool. This does not mean trying to swim! Stay in the shallow water and work on nice slow arms strokes. This can speed up healing tremendously. Being in the zero gravity environment of water is great for recovering from any shoulder surgery.

I love hearing success stories and you can email me at any time. My email is mstrtherapy@gmail.com. If you have a minute, please leave a quick amazon review of my book. It really helps and I would really appreciate it! I love honest reviews from people who used the treatments for a few months. Thank you

-William Prowse IV

Confused on which supplements to buy?

Check out my website to see my favorites!

Go Online and type this address into your web browser:

http://www.mstrtherapy.com/optimal-health-supplements.html

If you need relief from chronic injuries, check out:

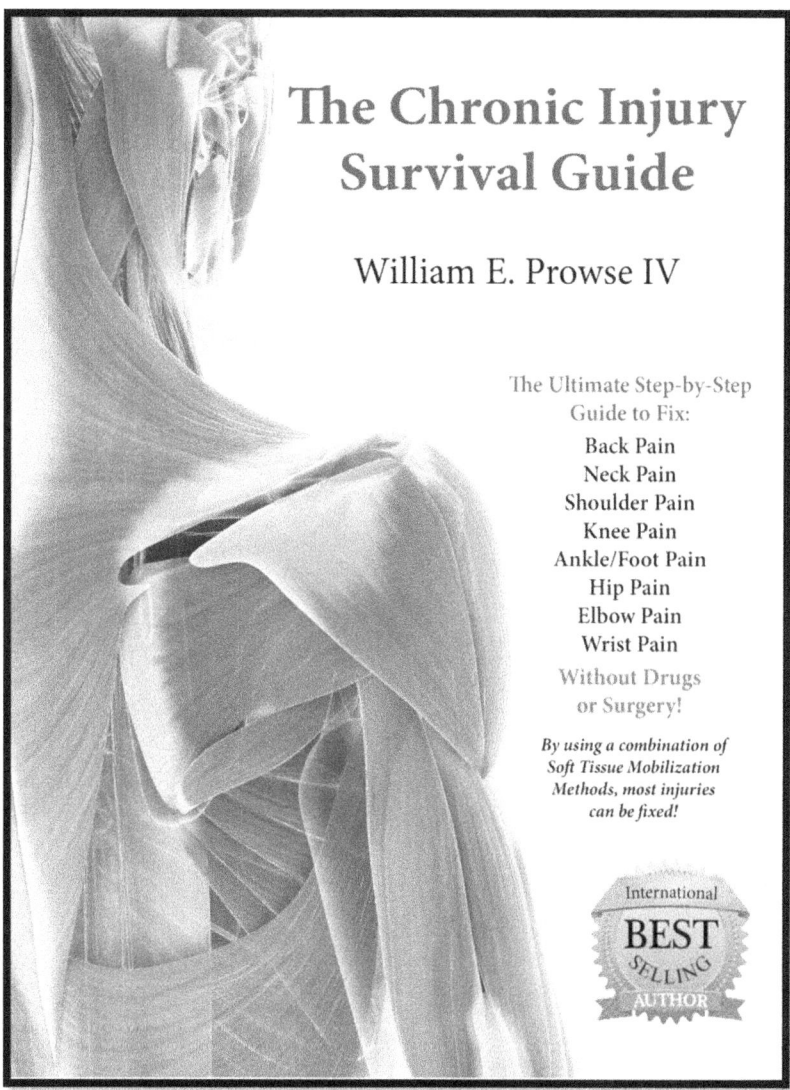

www.ingramcontent.com/pod-product-compliance
Lightning Source LLC
Chambersburg PA
CBHW080650180526
45168CB00008B/3369